Sirtfood Diet

Everything you need to get started. Easy
and Healthy Sirtfood Diet Recipes for
Weight Loss

By

Adele Green

1

TABLE OF CONTENTS

INTRODUCTION 7

HOW TO LOSE WEIGHT WITH THE SIRTFOOD DIET 10

THE SIRTFOOD DIET EXPLAINED 13

PHASES OF THE DIET 19

PHASE 1 20

SIRT FOODS 35

SIRTUINS FILLED INGREDIENTS 37

Cocoa 37

Chili pepper 37

Coffee 38

Green tea 38

Red wine 38

Kale 38

Buckwheat 39

Celery 39

Medjoul Dates 39

Capers 40

Extra virgin olive oil 40

Rocket salad 40

Parsley 41

Red chicory *41*

Soy *41*

Red onion: *42*

Strawberries: *42*

Walnuts: *42*

Supplements *43*

SIRTFOOD DIET'S BENEFITS 44

RECIPES 46

CENTRIFUGED GREEN JUICE 46

CHICKEN WITH RED ONION AND KALE 47

TURKEY WITH CAULIFLOWER COUSCOUS 48

ORIENTAL PRAWNS WITH BUCKWHEAT 49

MISO AND TOFU WITH SESAME GLAZE AND SAUTÉED

VEGETABLES IN A PAN WITH GINGER AND CHILI 51

CAULIFLOWER COUSCOUS 52

TURKEY ESCALOPES WITH SAGE, PARSLEY, AND

CAPERS 54

CABBAGE AND RED ONION DAHL WITH BUCKWHEAT

.... 55

AROMATIC CHICKEN BREAST WITH KALE, RED ONION,

TOMATO SAUCE AND CHILI 57

BAKED TOFU WITH HARISSA 58

SIRT MUESLI 59

PAN-FRIED SALMON FILLET WITH CARAMELIZED

RADICCHIO SALAD, ROCKET AND CELERY LEAVES 60

TUSCAN STEWED BEANS.................................. 62

BUCKWHEAT TABBOULEH WITH STRAWBERRIES 63

BAKED COD MARINATED IN MISO WITH SAUTÉED
VEGETABLES AND SESAME 65

LENTILS, RED ONION AND TOMATOES SALAD 67

BEAN CREAM.. 69

BACON OMELET 70

CHICKEN WITH PARSLEY AND NUTS 71

CONCLUSIONS **73**

CRITICISMS.. 75

Introduction

Fasting-based diets have become very popular over the past few years. In fact, studies show that by fasting - that is, with moderate daily calorie restriction or by practicing a more radical, but less frequent, intermittent fast - you can expect to lose about 3 kg in six months and substantially reduce the risk of contracting certain diseases.

When we fast, the reduction of energy reserves activates the so-called "skinny gene", which causes several positive changes. The accumulation of fat stops and the body blocks normal growth processes and enters the "survival" mode. Fats are burned faster and the genes that repair and rejuvenate cells are activated. As a result, we lose weight and increase our resistance to diseases.

All this, however, has a price. Lower energy intake leads to hunger, irritability, exhaustion and loss of muscle mass. And this is a problem the main problem with fasting-based diets: when they are followed correctly, they work, but they make us feel so bad that we cannot repeat them. The question, then, is the following: is it possible to obtain the same results without having to impose that drastic drop in calories and, therefore, without suffering the negative consequences?

According to the Sirtfood Diet, it is. In fact, there is a skinny gene that, if activated properly, allows you to lose weight and gain health altogether. The singer Adele has lost 30 kilos in a year thanks to this philosophy: a program of two medical nutritionists, Aidan Goggins and Glen Matten, which is based on the introduction of some Sirt foods in our diet.

These are particularly nutrient-rich foods capable of activating the same skinny genes stimulated by fasting. These genes are called sirtuins and considered to be super regulators of metabolism so as to influence our ability to burn fat.

How to lose weight with the Sirtfood Diet

Singer Adele has confirmed that she has lost 30 kilos in just one year. The secret? Apparently, it's all thanks to the Sirtfood Diet. It was revealed by the singer herself through international media, such as the Daily Mail and the New York Post.

The Sirtfood Diet is not the classic fasting diet: Adele is the living proof of this, given the splendid shape in which was at her appointments with her fans. It is, in fact, a diet that leaves room for both cheese and red wine as well as chocolate, in the right proportions, and of course under the supervision of a specialist doctor, who knows how to evaluate your health and recommend the most suitable diet to lose weight safely.

Many were the media that underlined the substantial weight loss of the singer Adele who admitted, how the decision to lose weight did not depend on the acceptance of herself as much as the difficulty of using her voice to the fullest.

Adele praised the Sirtfood Diet, which made her lose 30 kilos without much effort (although in reality, she admitted via Instagram that she had never struggled as much in physical activity as when preparing for her tour). She also said that the beauty of Sirt foods is that many of them are already on our table every day. They are accessible and can be easily integrated into our diet.

Although being thinner was not her priority (the singer has always had an excellent relationship with her body), she wanted to review her eating habits to get back in shape, but also (or better above all) to feel good about herself.

Furthermore, the Sirtfood Diet had come back on the news because it was Pippa Middleton's choice to get back into shape quickly before her wedding with the millionaire James Matthews that was celebrated on May 20, 2017.

Pippa Middleton would have tested the concrete benefits of this hunger-free regime by eating the ingredients of the Sirtfood Diet prepared by nutritionists Aidan Goggins and Glen Matten with gusto. Nothing to do with the Dukan, diet followed by sister Kate before marrying Prince William, one of the many fasting diets that currently exist.

The Sirtfood Diet explained

The Sirtfood Diet, also called the skinny gene-diet, is the result of the studies of the two nutritionists Aidan Goggings and Glenn Matten. Their food program, published in a volume that explains its principles and functioning, has attracted the attention of VIPs and sportsmen. Its effectiveness is based on the consumption of foods that stimulate sirtuins. As the creators of the diet of the moment explain, it is a family of genes present in each of us. They affect the ability to burn fat in addition to mood and the mechanisms that regulate longevity. It is no coincidence that they are also called "super metabolic regulators." Recent studies have shown that there are a number of foods that can stimulate sirtuins. Their consumption would, therefore, allow them to activate the metabolism and lose weight without having to undergo extreme diets.

What makes the Sirtfood Diet different from the others is its "inclusion" philosophy. In fact, it is not based on the total or partial exclusion of some foods from your diet. Rather, it suggests which foods should be added to lose weight more easily. In this way, you will no longer have to undergo excessive deprivation or exhausting willpower. And you won't have to resort to expensive supplements or products with mysterious components. By eating a balanced diet and supporting it, if desired, with proper physical activity, according to the two nutritionists, you can lose about 3.5 kilos in a week.

Sirt foods are particularly rich in special nutrients, capable of activating the same genes of thinness stimulated by fasting. These genes are sirtuins. They became famous thanks to an important study conducted in 2003, during which scientists analyzed a particular substance, resveratrol, present in the peel of black grapes, red wine, and yeast, which would produce the same effects of calorie restriction without need to decrease your daily calories intake. Later, researchers found that other substances in red wine had a similar effect, which would explain the benefits of consuming this drink and why those who consume it get less fat.

This naturally stimulated the search for other foods containing a high concentration of these nutrients, capable of producing such a beneficial effect on the body, and studies gradually discovered several. If some are almost unknown, such as lovage, an herb that is by now very little used in cooking, the great majority is represented by well-known and widely used foods, such as extra virgin olive oil, red onions, parsley, chili, kale, strawberries, capers, tofu, cocoa, green tea, and even coffee.

After the discovery in 2003, the enthusiasm for the benefits of Sort's food skyrocketed. Studies revealed that these foods don't just mimic the effects of calorie restriction. They also act as super regulators of the entire metabolism: they burn fat, increase muscle mass, and improve the health of our cells. The world of medical research was close to the most important nutritional discovery of the century. Unfortunately, a mistake was made: the pharmaceutical industry invested hundreds of millions of pounds in an attempt to turn Sirt foods into a sort of miracle pill, and the diet took a back seat. The Sirtfood Diet, however, does not share this pharmaceutical approach, which seeks (so far without result) to concentrate the benefits of these complex nutrients of plant origin into a single drug. Instead of waiting for the pharmaceutical industry to transform the nutrients of the foods we eat into a miraculous product (which may not work anyway), the Sirtfood Diet consists of eating these substances in their natural form that of food, to take full advantage of them. This is the basis of the pilot experiment of the Sirtfood Diet, with which the creators intended to create a diet containing the richest sources of Sirt foods and observe their effects.

During their studies, Glen Matten and Aidan Goggins discovered that the best Sirt foods are consumed regularly by populations who boast the lowest incidence of diseases and obesity in the world.

The Kuna Indians, in the American continent, seem immune from hypertension and with very low levels of obesity, diabetes, cancer, and early death thanks to the intake of cocoa, excellent Sirt food. In Okinawa, Japan, Sirt food, dry physique, and longevity go hand in hand. In India, the passion for spicy foods, especially turmeric, gives good results in the fight against cancer. And in the traditional Mediterranean diet, which the rest of the western world envies, obesity is contained, and chronic diseases are the exception, not the norm. Extra virgin olive oil, wild green leafy vegetables, dried fruit, berries, red wine, dates, and aromatic herbs are all effective Sirt foods, and they are all present in the Mediterranean diet. The scientific world has had to surrender to the evidence: it seems that the Mediterranean diet is more effective than reducing calories to lose weight and more effective than drugs to eliminate diseases.

Although Sirt foods are not a mainstay of nutrition in most of the western world today, the situation was quite different in the past. They were a basic element, and if many have become rare and others have even disappeared, it is definitely possible to reverse the course of this.

The good news is that you don't have to be a top athlete, and not even sporty, to enjoy the same benefits. We took advantage of everything we learned about Sirt foods thanks to the pilot study by KX and the work done with sportsmen, and we adapted it to create a diet suitable for anyone who wants to lose weight while improving health.

It is not necessary to practice unsustainable fasting or to undergo endless sessions in the gym (although, of course, practicing a little physical activity would be good for you). It is not an expensive diet nor will it waste your time, and all the foods recommended in the diet are readily available. The only accessory you will need is an extractor or centrifuge. Unlike other diets, which tell you what to eliminate, this diet tells you what to eat.

Phases of the diet

Phase 1 of the diet is the one that produces the greatest results. Over the course of seven days, you will follow a simple method in order to lose 3.5 kg. Following, you will find a step-by-step guide, complete with menus and recipes.

During the first three days, the intake of calories will have to be limited to one thousand per day at most. Basically, you can have three green juices and a solid meal, all based on Sirt foods. From day 4 to 7, the daily calories will become fifteen hundred. Every day you will eat two green juices and two solid Sirt meals. By the end of the seven days, you should have lost, on average, 3.5 kilos.

Despite the reduction in calories, the participants do not feel hungry, and the calorie limit is an indication rather than a goal. Even in the most intensive phase, calorie restriction is not as drastic as in many other regimes. Sirt foods have a naturally satiating effect so that many of you will feel pleasantly full and satisfied.

Phase 2 is the maintenance phase and lasts 14 days: during this period, although the main objective is not the reduction of calories, you will consolidate weight loss and continue to lose weight. The secret to succeeding at this stage lies in continuing to eat Sirt foods in abundance; following the program that we will provide you with relative recipes will facilitate you. During those two weeks, you will consume three balanced and rich Sirt foods per day and a green Sirt juice.

Phase 1

Monday: 3 green juices

- Breakfast: water + tea or espresso + a cup of green juice;
- Lunch: green juice
- Snack: a square of dark chocolate;
- Dinner: Sirt meal
- After dinner: a square of dark chocolate.

Drink the juices at three distinct times of the day (for example, in the morning as soon as you wake up, mid-morning and mid-afternoon) and choose the normal or vegan dish: pan-fried oriental prawns with buckwheat spaghetti or miso and tofu with sesame glaze and sautéed vegetables (vegan dish)

Tuesday: 3 green juices

- Breakfast: water + tea or espresso + a cup of green juice
- Lunch: 2 green juices before dinner;
- Snack: a square of dark chocolate;
- Dinner: Sirt meal
- After dinner: a square of dark chocolate.

Welcome to day 2 of the Sirtfood Diet. The formula is identical to that of the first day, and the only thing that changes is the solid meal. Today you will also have dark chocolate, and the same goes for tomorrow. This food is so wonderful that we don't need an excuse to eat it.

To earn the title of a "Sirt food", chocolate must be at least 85 percent cocoa. And even among the various types of chocolate with this percentage, not all of them are the same. Often this product is treated with an alkalizing agent (this is the so-called "Dutch process") to reduce its acidity and give it a darker color. Unfortunately, this process greatly reduces the flavonoids activating sirtuins, compromising their health benefits. Lindt Excellence 85% chocolate, is not subjected to the Dutch process and is therefore often recommended.

On day 2, capers are also included in the menu. Despite what many may think, they are not fruits, but buds that grow in Mediterranean countries and are picked by hand. They are fantastic Sirt foods because they are very rich in the nutrients kaempferol and quercetin. From the point of view of flavour, they are tiny concentrates of taste. If you've never used them, don't feel intimidated. You will see, they will taste amazingly if combined with the right ingredients, and they will give an unmistakable and inimitable aroma to your dishes.

On the second day, you will intake: 3 green Sirt juices and one solid meal (normal or vegan).

Drink the juices at three distinct times of the day (for example, when you wake up in the morning, mid-morning and mid-afternoon) and choose either the normal or the vegan dish:

Turkey escalope with capers, parsley, and sage on spiced cauliflower couscous or curly kale and red onion dahl with buckwheat (vegan dish)

Wednesday: 3 green juices

- Breakfast: water + tea or espresso + a cup of green juice
- Lunch: 2 green juices before dinner;
- Snack: a square of dark chocolate;
- Dinner: Sirt meal
- After dinner: a square of dark chocolate.

You are now on the third day, and even if the format is once again identical to that of days 1 and 2, so the time has come to flavor everything with a fundamental ingredient. For thousands of years, chili has been a fundamental element of the gastronomic experiences of the whole world.

As for the effects on health, we have already seen that its spiciness is perfect for activating sirtuins and stimulating the metabolism. The applications of chili are endless, and therefore represent an easy way to consume a Sirt food regularly. Aware that not everyone loves spicy or spicy food, we recommend that you at least try to use small quantities, especially since it has been shown that those who eat spicy at least three times a week have a mortality rate of 14 percent lower than those who eat spicy foods less than once a week.

If you are not a big expert of chili, we recommend the Bird's Eye (sometimes called Thai chili), because it is the best for sirtuins.

This is the last day you will consume three green juices a day; tomorrow, you will switch to two. We, therefore, take this opportunity to browse other drinks that you can have during the diet. We all know that green tea is good for health, and water is naturally very good, but what about coffee? More than half of people drink at least one coffee a day, but always with a trace of guilt because some say that it is a vice and an unhealthy habit. This is absolutely untrue; studies show that coffee is a real treasure trove of beneficial plant substances. That's why coffee drinkers run the least risk of getting diabetes, certain forms of cancer, and neurodegenerative diseases.

Furthermore, not only is coffee, not a toxin, it protects the liver and makes it even healthier!

On the third day, you will intake 3 green Sirt juices and 1 one solid meal (normal or vegan, see below).

Drink the juices at three distinct times of the day (for example, in the morning as soon as you wake up, mid-morning and mid-afternoon) and choose the normal or vegan dish: aromatic chicken breast with kale, red onion, tomato sauce, and chili or baked tofu with harissa on spiced cauliflower couscous (vegan dish)

Thursday: 3 green juices

- Breakfast: water + tea or espresso + a cup of green juice;
- Lunch: Sirt food;
- Snack: 1 green juice before dinner
- Dinner: Sirt food

The fourth day of the Sirtfood Diet has arrived, and you are halfway through your journey to a leaner and healthier body. The big change from the previous three days is that you will only drink two juices instead of three and that you will have two solid meals instead of one.

This means that on the fourth day and the upcoming ones, you will have two green juices and two solid meals, all delicious and rich in Sirt foods. The inclusion of Medjoul dates in a list of foods that promote weight loss and good health may seem surprising. Especially when you think they contain 66 percent sugar.

Sugar has no stimulating properties towards sirtuins. On the contrary, it has well-known links with obesity, heart disease, and diabetes; in short, just at the antipodes of the objectives, we aim to. But industrially refined and processed sugar is very different from the sugar present in a food that also contains sirtuin-activating polyphenols: the Medjoul dates. Unlike normal sugar, these dates, consumed in moderation, do not increase the level of glucose in the blood.

Today we will also integrate chicory into meals. Like with onion, red chicory is better in this case too, but endive, its close relative, is also a Sirt food. If you are looking for ideas on the use of these salads, combine them with other varieties and season them with olive oil:

they will give a pungent flavor to milder leaves.

On the fourth day, you will intake: 2 green Sirt juices, 2 solid meals (normal or vegan)

Drink the juices at different times of the day (for example the first in the morning as soon as you wake up or in the middle of the morning, the second in the middle of the afternoon) and choose the normal or vegan dishes: muesli Sirt, pan-fried salmon fillet with caramelized chicory, rocket salad, and celery leaves or muesli Sirt and Tuscan stewed beans (vegan dish)

Friday: 2 green juices

• Breakfast: water + tea or espresso + a cup of green juice

- Lunch: Sirt food
- Snack: a green juice before dinner;
- Dinner: Sirt food

You have reached the fifth day, and the time has come to add fruits. Due to its high sugar content, fruits have been the subject of bad publicity. This does not apply to berries.

Strawberries have a very low sugar content: one teaspoon per 100 grams. They also have an excellent effect on how the body processes simple sugars.

Scientists have found that if we add strawberries to simple sugars, this causes a reduction in insulin demand, and therefore transforms food into a machine that releases energy for a long time. Strawberries are, therefore, a perfect element in diets that will help you lose weight and get back in shape. They are also delicious and extremely versatile, as you will discover in the Sirt version of the fresh and light Middle Eastern tabbouleh.

Miso, made from fermented soy, is a traditional Japanese dish. Miso contains a strong umami taste, a real explosion for the taste buds. In our modern society, we know better monosodium glutamate, artificially created to reproduce the same flavor. Needless to say, it is far preferable to derive that magical umami flavor from traditional and natural food, full of beneficial substances. It is found in the form of a paste in all good supermarkets and healthy food stores and should be present in every kitchen to give a touch of taste to many different dishes.

Since umami flavors enhance each other, miso is perfectly associated with other tasty/umami foods, especially when it comes to cooked proteins, as you will discover today in the very tasty, fast and easy dishes you will eat.

On the fifth day, you will intake 2 green Sirt juices and 2 solid meals (normal or vegan).

Drink the juices at different times of the day (for example the first in the morning as soon as you wake up or in the middle of the morning, the second in the middle of the afternoon) and choose the normal or vegan dishes: buckwheat Tabbouleh with strawberries, baked cod marinated in miso with sautéed vegetables and sesame or buckwheat and strawberry Tabbouleh (vegan dish), soba (buckwheat noodles) in a miso broth with tofu, celery, and kale (vegan dish).

Saturday: 2 green juices

- Breakfast: water + tea or espresso + a cup of green juice

- Lunch: Sirt food
- Snack: a green juice before dinner;
- Dinner: Sirt food

There are no Sirt foods better than olive oil and red wine. Virgin olive oil is obtained from the fruit only by mechanical means, in conditions that do not deteriorate it, so that you can be sure of its quality and polyphenol content. "Extra virgin" oil is that of the first pressing ("virgin" is the result of the second) and therefore has more flavor and better quality: this is what we strongly recommend you to use when cooking.

No Sirt menu would be complete without red wine, one of the cornerstones of the diet. It contains the activators of resveratrol and piceatannol sirtuins, which probably explain the longevity and slenderness associated with the traditional French way of life, and which are at the origin of the enthusiasm unleashed by Sirt foods.

Of course, wine contains alcohol, so it should be consumed in moderation. Fortunately, resveratrol can withstand heat well, and therefore can be used in the kitchen. Pinot

Noir is many people's favorite grape variety because it contains much more resveratrol than most of the others.

On the sixth day, you will assume 2 green Sirt juices and 2 solid meals (normal or vegan).

Drink the juices at different times of the day (for example, the first in the morning as soon as you wake up or in the middle of the morning, the second in the middle of the afternoon) and choose the normal or vegan dishes: Super Sirt salad and grilled beef fillet with red wine sauce, onion rings, garlic curly kale and roasted potatoes with aromatic herbs or

super lentil Sirt salad (vegan dish) and mole sauce of red beans with roasted potato (vegan dish).

Sunday: 2 green juices

- Breakfast: a bowl of Sirt Muesli + a cup of green juice
- Lunch: Sirt food
- Snack: a cup of green juice;
- dinner: Sirt food

The seventh day is the last of phase 1 of the diet. Instead of considering it as an end, see it as a beginning, because you are about to embark on a new life, in which Sirt foods will play a central role in your nutrition. Today's menu is a perfect example of how easy it is to integrate them in abundance into your daily diet. Just take your favorite dishes and, with a pinch of creativity, you will turn them into a Sirt banquet.

Walnuts are excellent Sirt food because they contradict current opinions. They have high fat content and many calories, yet it has been shown that they contribute to reducing weight and metabolic diseases, all thanks to the activation of sirtuins. They are also a versatile ingredient, excellent in baked dishes, in salads and as a snack, alone.

Pesto is becoming an irreplaceable ingredient in the kitchen because it is tasty and allows you to give personality to even the simplest dishes. The traditional one is made with basil and pine nuts, but you can try an alternative one with parsley and walnuts. The result is delicious and rich in Sirt foods.

We can apply the same reasoning to an easy-to-prepare dish, such as an omelet. The dish has to be the typical recipe appreciated by the whole family, and simple to transform into a Sirt dish with a few little tricks. In our recipe, we use bacon. Why? Simply because it fits perfectly. The Sirtfood Diet tells us what to include, not what to exclude, and this allows us to change our long-term eating habits. After all, isn't that the secret to not getting back the lost pounds and staying healthy?

On the seventh day, you will assume 2 green Sirt juices; 2 solid meals (normal or vegan).

Drink the juices at different times of the day (for example the first in the morning as soon as you wake up or in the middle of the morning, the second in the middle of the afternoon) and choose the normal or vegan dishes: Sirt omelet Sirt and baked chicken breast with walnut and parsley pesto and red onion salad or Walldorf salad (vegan dish) and baked aubergine wedges with walnut and parsley pesto and tomato salad (vegan dish).

During the second phase, there are no calorie restrictions but indications on which Sirt foods must be eaten to consolidate weight loss and not run the risk of getting the lost kilograms back.

Sirt foods

The skinny gene-diet is not difficult to follow and is divided into two phases. The first phase lasts 7 days and is more restrictive and difficult, especially for the first 3 days. To be able to lose 3 kg per week as promised by this diet, it is advisable, initially, not to exceed 1000 calories per day during the first 3 days, drinking 3 green juices based on sirtuin-rich foods and eating only one solid meal of your choice, prepared using the ingredients indicated above.

From the 4th to the 7th day, instead, you can ingest 1500 calories per day by consuming three green juices and two solid meals composed of foods rich in sirtuins.

Generally, you can eat foods that are high in protein and low in fat. Among the meat-based recipes, you can choose for example Chicken with red onion and black cabbage, Turkey with cauliflower couscous, turkey escalope with capers and parsley. For fish dishes, sautéed salmon fillet, sautéed prawns, or baked marinated cod are fine.

Recipes of side dishes, light and tasty, can be prepared with beans, lentils, aubergines cut into wedges, and cooked in the oven, Walldorf salad, or red onions. And as for dessert, you can eat delicious and healthy strawberries, with a very high content of sirtuins. Plus, remember that 15-20 g of dark chocolate are allowed every day.

The green juice is an important part of the diet, because it has the ability to cleanse and detoxify, and will be the protagonist in the first week of the Sirt program.

Sirt foods are particularly rich in special nutrients of plant origin recently discovered, which, stimulated by fasting, activate the genes of thinness.

The foods suggested in the Sirtfood Diet are fresh, genuine and easily available, such as extra virgin olive oil, dark chocolate, citrus fruits, strawberries, apples, cabbage, celery, spinach, buckwheat, blueberries, nuts, soya beans, rocket salad, red onion, coffee, green tea**, red wine, chili pepper***, tofu, turmeric, and dates.

In addition, combined with each other or with other foods, they allow you to create very tasty dishes.

Sirtuins filled ingredients

Cocoa

Yes, to chocolate, but not any type! It must be dark chocolate and present at least 85% of cocoa. Useful above all to appease hunger, therefore mostly used as a snack.

Lindt Excellence 85%, which retains a good percentage of flavonoids, and Rowntree's cocoa powder are the most highly recommended.

Chili pepper***

To make your dishes spicier, use Bird's Eye chili (also called Thai chili), very rich in sirtuin. You can use it at least three times a week.

Warning! Compared to normal chili, the Bird's Eye is much spicier; to get used to it, in the beginning, use only half of what is indicated in the recipe, eliminating the seeds, which are very spicy.

Coffee

You can drink 3-4 cups of coffee a day being careful not to overdo it with sugar, and avoid adding milk.

Green tea**

Known because it is so good for our body, green tea contributes to the loss of fat, preserving your muscles. Choose the Matcha variety and drink it with the addition of a little lemon juice, which increases the absorption of the nourishing activators of sirtuins.

Red wine

The research that gave rise to the Sirtfood Diet started with red wine. The first Sirt slimming element discovered, in fact, is resveratrol, present in black grape's skin and red wine. It appears that this nutrient attacks fat cells. In addition, red wine contains piceatannol, associated with longevity.

Kale

Kale is a suitable food for every diet. It is cheap and easy to find. It contains in large quantities two nutrients that activate sirtuins:

kaempferol and quercetin, which act in synergy to prevent the formation of fat.

Buckwheat

This " pseudo-cereal " is very popular in Japan and is a nutritious and highly satiating food, properties on which this type of nutrition focuses. So yes, to seeds, flakes, and buckwheat pasta.

Celery

The nutritive parts of celery, used for millennia, also as a medicinal plant, are the heart and the leaves: here, in fact, the activators of the sirtuins are contained, which are apigenin and luteolin. A tip: if you can, choose the green one instead of the white one.

Medjoul Dates

Although dates are composed of 66% sugar, they also contain " good " polyphenols that activate sirtuins. So, unlike normal sugars, date nutrients do not increase the amount of glucose in the blood, but their consumption seems instead associated with a lower incidence of diabetes and heart disease.

However, always remember to eat them in moderation!

Capers

The caper plant is widespread in Mediterranean countries, and its fruits are highly appreciated for their " concentrate of taste " capable of reviving even the most anonymous dishes. Taste aside, capers are also very rich in active-sirtuin nutrients, such as kaempferol and quercetin.

Extra virgin olive oil

Good and healthy, the extra virgin olive oil, obtained from the first pressing of the olives, is a perfect seasoning and tastes very good both on vegetables and on bread! Rich in polyphenols, vitamin E and " good " fatty acids, it will be your heart and youth's best friend, thanks to its antioxidant properties.

Rocket salad

Arugula is a vegetable rich in nutrients that activate the metabolism, such as quercetin and kaempferol. Its peppery and decisive flavor can embellish many recipes, and it especially goes with olive oil.

A curiosity: they began to cultivate it for the first time in ancient Rome, where it seems it was very appreciated for its aphrodisiac qualities.

Parsley

It is a basic ingredient to enrich practically any dish and a lot of sauces. It tastes fresh and is used to relieve itching and toothache. The Sirtfood Diet appreciates it above all because it is one of the foods with the highest concentration of apigenin, an activator of sirtuins.

Red chicory

It can be consumed within this diet in large quantities, both alone and accompanied by other Sirt foods. A greedy idea? Caramelized red chicory salad with celery leaves.

Soy

In addition to its beneficial properties, associated with the activating action of daidzein and formononetin, soy has an unmistakable flavor that makes every dish tastier.

Soy sauce, soy yogurt, and miso, a traditional Japanese dish based on salt-fermented soybeans, are all amazing. Red (saltier) and brown miso, are the most suitable qualities to prepare Sirt recipes

Red onion:

Tasty and rich in quercetin, which activates the metabolism. It is important to peel it and consume it raw to keep the nutrients active so that they can act better on sirtuins.

Strawberries:

They have few sugars, are delicious and will also make you lose weight because they are the main source of fisetin, a sirtuin activator.

Walnuts:

They are rich in fats and very caloric, yet, according to Sirt nutritionists, this food should promote weight loss by also fighting metabolic diseases. In addition, walnuts contain a lot of minerals, which are extremely useful for the body, such as magnesium, zinc, copper, calcium, and iron. An idea for a first course? Try an alternative pesto with walnuts and parsley.

Supplements

In the presence of food deficiencies, it may be appropriate to restore the body's balance by providing it with an extra dose of those nutrients that are missing or are in short supply in our everyday diet. However, remember that supplements shouldn't be eaten "for fun", so it is always advisable to seek medical advice before taking any product, even if it is as natural as it comes.

Sirtfood Diet's benefits

The best thing about this diet is that you are not always forced to starve yourself. Phase 1 and Phase 2 can be repeated from time to time to lose fat if necessary. For someone, it might be essential to repeat them every three months, while for someone other people, it will be enough to repeat it once a year. The rest of the time, you are free to live your life, skinnier, and healthier than before, continuing to enjoy the benefits of a diet rich in Sirt foods. In fact, these foods have a universal application and can be incorporated in any type of dietary regime: vegan, gluten-free, low in carbohydrates, intermittent fasting, and so on. Incorporating significant quantities of Sirt foods will enhance the weight loss and health benefits of all those approaches.

The secret of success is to achieve results that will last a lifetime, and the Sirtfood Diet is truly exceptional in that sense. When you will have assimilated the cornerstones of a balanced diet and the correct use of supplements, and you have discovered the practical tips to consume even more Sirt foods, you will be ready to benefit from them for the rest of your life.

Here is a list of the benefits of the Sirtfood Diet:

- promotes fat loss, not muscle loss;
- you will not regain weight after the end of the diet;
- you will look better; you will feel better, and you will have more energy;
- you will avoid fasting and feeling hungry;
- you will not have to undergo exhausting physical exercises;
- This diet promotes a longer, healthier life and keeps diseases away.

The benefits of the Sirtfood Diet are many, besides obviously that of slimming. Activators of sirtuins would lead to a noticeable muscle building, decreased appetite, and improved memory. In addition, the Sirtfood Diet normalizes the level of sugar in the blood and is able to cleanse the cells from the accumulation of harmful free radicals.

Recipes

Centrifuged green juice

Ingredients

Green juice has the ability to purify and satiate and will be the protagonist of the first week of the food plan. To prepare it you need:

- 75 g of kale
- 30 g of rocket salad
- 5 g of parsley
- 150 g of green celery with the leaves
- 1/2 green apple
- 1/2 lemon juice
- 1/2 teaspoon of matcha tea

Preparation

Centrifuge the kale, rocket salad and parsley; add grated celery and apple; enrich with half a squeezed lemon and half a teaspoon of matcha tea. Drink immediately so as not to lose the beneficial effects of vegetables and not keep it in the fridge. It should always be prepared when consuming it.

Chicken with red onion and kale

Ingredients

- 120 g chicken breast
- 130 g of tomatoes
- 1 Bird's Eye chili
- 1 tablespoon of capers
- 5 g of parsley
- lemon juice
- 2 teaspoons of extra virgin olive oil
- 2 teaspoons of turmeric
- 50 g of kale
- 20 g of red onion
- 1 teaspoon fresh ginger
- 50 g of buckwheat

Preparation

Marinate the chicken breast for 10 minutes with 1/4 of lemon juice, 1 teaspoon of extra virgin olive oil and 1 teaspoon of turmeric powder. Cut 130 g of tomatoes into chunks, remove the inside, season with the chili pepper, 1 tablespoon of capers, 1 teaspoon of turmeric and one of extra virgin olive oil, 1/4 lemon juice and 5 g of chopped parsley.

Cook the drained chicken breast on high heat for one minute per side and then put it in the oven for about 10 minutes, at 220 °. Let it rest covered by an aluminum foil. Steam the minced kale for 5 minutes, in a pan fry the red onion, a teaspoon of grated fresh ginger and a teaspoon of extra virgin olive oil; add the boiled cabbage and leave to flavor for one minute on the fire, boil the buckwheat with the turmeric, drain and serve with the chicken, tomatoes and chopped kale.

Turkey with Cauliflower Couscous

Ingredients

- 150 g of turkey
- 150 g of cauliflower
- 40 g of red onion
- 1 teaspoon fresh ginger
- 1 pepper Bird's Eye
- 1 clove of garlic
- 3 tablespoons of extra virgin olive oil
- 2 teaspoons of turmeric
- 30 g of dried tomatoes
- 10 g parsley
- dried sage to taste
- 1 tablespoon of capers

- 1/4 of fresh lemon juice

Preparation

Blend the raw cauliflower tops and cook them in a teaspoon of extra virgin olive oil, garlic, red onion, chili pepper, ginger, and a teaspoon of turmeric.

Leave to flavor on the fire for a minute, then add the chopped sun-dried tomatoes and 5 g of parsley. Season the turkey slice with a teaspoon of extra virgin olive oil, the dried sage and cook it in another teaspoon of extra virgin olive oil. Once ready, season with a tablespoon of capers, 1/4 of lemon juice, 5 g of parsley, a tablespoon of water and add the cauliflower.

Oriental prawns with buckwheat

Ingredients

- •150g of shrimps
- 1 spoon of turmeric
- 1 spoon of extra-virgin oil
- 75 gr of grain spaghetti
- Cooking water
- Salt

- 1 clove of garlic
- Bird's Eye chili
- 1 spoon of ginger
- red onion
- 40 g of celery
- 75 g of green beans
- 50 g of kale
- broth

Preparation

Cook for 2-3 minutes the peeled prawns with 1 teaspoon of tamari and 1 teaspoon of

extra virgin olive oil. Boil the buckwheat noodles in salt-free water, drain and set aside.

Fry with another teaspoon of extra virgin olive oil, 1 clove of garlic, 1 Bird's Eye chili and 1 teaspoon of finely chopped fresh ginger, 20 g of red onion and 40 g of sliced celery, 75 g of

chopped green beans, 50 g of curly kale roughly chopped.

Add 100 ml of broth and bring to a boil, letting it simmer until the vegetables are cooked and soft. Add the prawns, spaghetti, and 5 g of celery leaves, bring to the boil, and serve.

Miso and tofu with sesame glaze and sautéed vegetables in a pan with ginger and chili

Ingredients

- 2 teaspoons of extra virgin olive oil
- 200 g of mushrooms (enoki or champignon)
- ½ carrot, peeled and cut into julienne strips
- 1 red chili pepper, sliced
- 1 tablespoon of fresh ginger
- •cabbage or spinach
- onion
- miso paste
- 125 g of tofu

Preparation

Heat the oil in a large pan and add the mushrooms and carrot. Quickly cook the vegetables for a minute or as long as they are tender, then add the chili and ginger and cook for another 10 seconds.

Add the cabbage or spinach and ì onions in the pan and cook until the leaves are slightly wilted. Remove them from the pans and divide them into two bowls.

Bring 700 ml of water to the boiling point in a large saucepan. In a small bowl, mix the miso with a couple of teaspoons of water and add it to the pot. Stir to mix and still incorporate miso if necessary. Divide the drained and diced tofu into the bowls and cover with the miso broth. Add tamari or soy sauce and serve immediately.

Cauliflower couscous

Ingredients

- 800 g cauliflower
- 7 dried tomatoes
- 1 tablespoon of capers
- 1 anchovy in oil
- 2 tablespoons of pitted Taggiasca olives
- 1 clove of garlic
- 200 g of marinated anchovies
- fresh oregano
- extra virgin olive oil

Preparation

To prepare the cauliflower couscous, remove the leaves and remove the florets. Rinse the couscous under running freshwater, dab them with kitchen paper to dry them and blend them, a little at a time, in a food processor and transfer the granules obtained in a clean bowl.

Let the dried tomatoes soak in lukewarm water for half an hour, then squeeze them, dab them with paper towels and cut them into thin strips. Drain the capers and chop half of them with a knife. Coarsely chop also half of the olives. Peel the garlic and mash it with the palm of your hand. In a large pan, heat a little oil. Fry the garlic with the capers (chopped and whole), the anchovy and the chopped olives. Also, add the sliced tomatoes over high heat.

Pour the cauliflower grains and stir in with a little water (about half a glass: the cauliflower must remain crunchy), always on high heat , and stir. Add salt, turn off the heat and add the anchovies marinated in fillets, the remaining olives, a few fresh oregano leaves and a round of raw oil.

Serve the cauliflower couscous hot or cold, depending on your taste.

Turkey escalopes with sage, parsley, and capers

Ingredients

- 8 slices of turkey
- Half white onion
- 1 large sprig of parsley
- A few fresh sage leaves or a nice pinch of the dried one
- Olive oil to taste
- Salt
- Capers
- Flour

Preparation

Cover the turkey slices with flour once at the time, shake them slightly to remove excess flour. Wash parsley, sage, and finely chop them with a knife, add the capers. Finely chop the onion, heat up 2 tablespoons of oil in a pan, add the onion, fry 1 minute, add 2 tablespoons of water, lower the heat, cover and cook the onion, add 3 tablespoons of oil, raise the heat, put on the heat the slices of turkey in the pan, brown them on both sides, salt.

One minute before turning off the heat, sprinkle the slices with the chopped sage and parsley with capers. Serve with the sauce made from the pan.

Cabbage and red onion dahl with buckwheat

Ingredients

- 250 gr hulled buckwheat
- 300 gr curly cabbage
- Vegetable broth
- 130 gr 1 Tomato pulp
- 2 spoons of extra virgin olive oil
- Red onion
- Basil
- Chopped chili pepper
- 800 gr of Water
- Pepper
- Salt

Preparation

Pour the water into a pot, add the oil and, on the fire, wait until it boils and add the broth. Then turn off the heat. Meanwhile, wash the cauliflower, cut the florets into small pieces and drain them. Chop the shallot finely enough. Pour the buckwheat in a colander and rinse it under running water.

In another saucepan (large) pour two full spoons of oil, add the chopped shallot, the mince for sautéing and fry it on a soft flame, often mixing to prevent it from sticking to the pot. When the onion is transparent and dried, add the buckwheat and toast it for a few minutes, mixing without letting it stick to the bottom of the pot. Then add the tomato pulp, broth, chopped basil, chopped red pepper, and mix, then add the cauliflower florets.

Cook the Buckwheat and cauliflower soup for 30 minutes, covering the pan with a lid and on low heat, occasionally stirring so as not to stick the buckwheat to the pan. If necessary, season with salt. After cooking, serve the buckwheat and cauliflower soup with freshly ground pepper. If you like (and if you are not vegan, vegetarian or lactose intolerant), you could also add some grated pecorino cheese. Your buckwheat and cauliflower soup are ready!

Aromatic chicken breast with kale, red onion, tomato sauce and chili

Ingredients

- 1 teaspoon aromatic herbs
- Chili pepper
- Aromatic chicken breast
- cabbage
- Red onion
- tomato sauce

Preparation

Boil the chicken. Peel, stick and wash the carrot. Wash the celery stick, then peel and wash the shallot. Cut the vegetables into chunks. Bring 2 liters of water to a boil with cabbage, red onion and tomato sauce. Simmer the broth for about 15 minutes. Soak the chicken breast for about 25 minutes in the aromatic broth. Turn off the heat and let it cool in the cooking liquid.

Arrange the chicken breast on a cutting board, remove the central bone and cartilage. Cut the 2 halves with a sharp knife into 1 cm thick slices. Put a few grains of pink pepper between two sheets of parchment paper and chop them with the meat mallet.

Divide the slices into individual plates and garnish each plate.

Serve with the sauce.

Baked tofu with harissa

Ingredients

- 400 gr Tofu (100gr per serving)
- 180 gr cherry tomatoes
- 10 gr capers in salt
- 2 g Oregano
- Extra virgin olive oil
- Fresh chili 250 g
- Garlic 4 cloves
- Fresh coriander in leaves 1 tbsp
- Coriander powder 1 tbsp
- Dried mint 1 tbsp
- Extra virgin olive oil to taste
- Salt up to 1 tbsp
- Caraway seeds 1 tbsp

Preparation

Cut the tofu into slices of 100gr each, cut the cherry tomatoes in half. Place each slice of tofu in the center of a 20x20cm large sheet of parchment paper and season it with cherry tomatoes, capers, olives, oregano, and EVO oil. Close the toffee paper and bake at 250 ° C for 15min.

To prepare the Harissa, remove the stalks from the chilies, wash them, cut them, remove the internal seeds, and leave them to soak in a little water for at least 1 hour. After the hour, drain and crush them together with the other ingredients, or put everything in a mixer, and add as much oil as needed to make a very thick cream. Put the mixture in a glass jar and cover the surface with oil, which will serve to preserve the Harissa.

Sirt Muesli

Ingredients

- Muesli
- Low-fat yogurt
- Puffed buckwheat
- Coconut flakes

- Dates
- 100 g of strawberries
- 10 g of dark chocolate

Preparation

Simply mix all the ingredients and serve!

Pan-fried salmon fillet with caramelized radicchio salad, rocket and celery leaves

Ingredients

- Salmon Slices of 150 g each
- 8 oranges
- 1 lemon
- black pepper
- salt to taste.
- extra-virgin olive oil
- Rosemary
- Chili
- Rocket salad
- Celery leaves
- 1 shallot
- 1 tablespoon of brown sugar
- 2 tablespoons of red wine
- extra virgin olive oil
- salt

Preparation

Preparing salmon in a pan is very simple, and just as fast, that's how to proceed: heat a drizzle of extra virgin olive oil in a pan. As soon as the oil is hot, put the salmon steaks in the pan, on the meaty side. Lightly incise the scaly part (the skin), and cook for about 1 minute with sustained heat. Then turn them over and cook them also on the skin side. Add the rosemary sprig to the pan and let it take flavor. Salt and pepper slightly and make sure that the skin becomes rusty.

Cook for about 2 minutes. While cooking, with the help of a spoon, takes the cooking liquid and pour it on the salmon steaks in order flavor the whole dish. Once the skin of the salmon steaks has turned golden brown and toasted, remove the pan from the heat. Cut the lemon, lime, and orange into wedges and serve the salmon steaks with freshly prepared citrus wedges, a few sprigs of dill and freshly crushed chili pepper.

To prepare the caramelized rocket salad in a pan, start by peeling the shallot and washing the rocket salad thoroughly. Continue taking a non-stick pan, pour a drizzle of olive oil on the bottom, put on the fire, and brown the shallot cut into thin strips for a few minutes. Continue adding the already washed and chopped rocket salad. Sauté the rocket salad for about ten minutes over high heat then, add the brown sugar, wild fennel, and red wine vinegar.

Leave to cook for another couple of minutes to reduce the liquid and caramelize the sugar. If necessary, adjust the flavor by adding a pinch of salt and a little more sugar or vinegar. Turn off the heat and let the rocket salad cool in the pan for a few moments before serving.

Tuscan Stewed Beans

Ingredients

- 1 dl Extra virgin olive oil
- Salt to taste
- Pepper as needed.
- 500 gr Cannellini beans
- Sage
- Garlic clove
- 2,5 l water

Preparation

Soak the beans for at least 12 hours before cooking. Pour the beans in a crockpot with water, a clove of garlic, sage, and a generous pinch of salt, adjust the flame as low as possible.

When the water is boiling, cover the pot, and continue cooking for at least 3 and a half hours, taking care that the flame remains very low, the beans in the pot must not move around.

Once you are done cooking, serve the beans with extra virgin olive oil, salt, and pepper on the table.

Buckwheat tabbouleh with strawberries

Ingredients

- buckwheat (broken) 100 g
- Turmeric powder 2 tsp
- Avocado 1
- Tomatoes 130 g
- Tropea red onions 40 g
- Medjoul dates (pitted) 50 g
- Parsley 50 g

- Strawberries 200 g
- 2 tablespoons extra virgin olive oil
- Lemon juice 1
- Rocket 50 g

Preparation

Heat up the water to cook the buckwheat.

When it boils, add turmeric and buckwheat. Be careful not to overcook it. It is good to leave, it "al dente." When cooked, drain the buckwheat and set aside to cool. Take a large bowl to spice the tabbouleh.

Cut the tomatoes into cubes and let them drain for a few minutes in a colander to remove the water.

On a cutting board, begin to finely chop the red onion, dates, and parsley and combine them with buckwheat.

Peel the avocado and cut it into small cubes and add it with the tomatoes to the buckwheat. Cut the strawberries into slices and gently add them to the rest of the ingredients. Add the chopped arugula, oil, and lemon juice. Mix all the ingredients and let the buckwheat tabbouleh take on extra flavor for an hour before serving it at the table.

Baked cod marinated in miso with sautéed vegetables and sesame

Ingredients

- 300-400g of fish fillets (Mackerel, Cod, etc.)
- 2 spoons of miso
- Vegetables
- sesame

Clean the fish fillets, rinse them and dry them well with kitchen paper and mix all the seasonings in a bowl. Spread the sauce on the fish fillets, put them in a plastic bag with zipping (food use) then leave them to marinate in the fridge overnight (*). To cook them, take the fish fillets from the bag, remove the sauce from the fillets using kitchen paper (because this sauce burns easily during cooking)

The fish fillet can be roasted in the oven or fried in a pan with a little olive oil.

In the case of the oven: grease the grill and arrange the fillets putting the side with the skin down, cook them at 200 ° C for about 8-10 minutes, then turn them and continue to roast for 8-10 minutes

In the case of the pan: spread a piece of parchment paper on the pan and arrange the fillets placing the side with the skin down. Cook them on medium heat for 3-4 minutes. After that, turn the fillets and cook over low heat together with the vegetables and sesame with lid for about 10 minutes.

Soba in a miso broth with tofu, celery, and kale

- 1 l of water
- 4 teaspoons of miso paste
- Noodles 160 g
- Celery stalk and leaves 100 g
- Tofu
- Kale
- Salt
- Pepper

To prepare the noodles soup, start cutting all the ingredients: then mix and cook the vegetables for about 15 minutes. Then add the water flush. Salt and pepper to taste, then to flavor the soup, grate the fresh ginger and cover with a lid to cook the soup over moderate heat for at least 20 minutes, stirring occasionally and adding more water if necessary (you will need to keep the liquid level just above the ingredients). After the necessary time, pour the noodles into the soup and cook for a few minutes (or for the time indicated on the package).

At this point, also add the miso paste previously diluted in a couple of spoonsful of warm water, but be careful not to boil the broth because the nutritional properties of the miso are altered.

Lentils, red onion and tomatoes salad

Ingredients

- Dried lentils 250 g
- Cherry tomatoes 10
- Fresh spring onion 1
- Chopped chives 2 tbsp
- Chili pepper 1
- Basil 12 leaves
- Extra virgin olive oil 6 tbsp
- White pepper to taste
- Salt to taste

Preparation

Boil the lentils in abundant salted water for about 20 minutes and turn off the heat when they are still crisp; if you want to soak the lentils the night before, the cooking time will be reduced by a few minutes. Drain the cooked lentils, and let them cool.

In the meantime, peel and finely chop the spring onion, chop the chives, cut the chili into small wheels and the cherry tomatoes into quarters, or into even smaller pieces. In a small bowl, create an emulsion with the oil, ground pepper, and salt.

Place the cold lentils in a large bowl: add the previously prepared ingredients, add the chili pepper, and the basil leaves chopped with your fingers (keep a few whole to garnish the lentil salad). Season with the oil emulsion and mix everything well, adjusting if necessary, with salt. Serve after decorating the lentil salad with a few fresh basil leaves.

Bean cream

Ingredients

- Dried black beans 200 g
- Onions 100 g
- Salt to taste
- Cumin powder the tip of 1 tsp
- Coriander powder the tip of 1 tsp
- Black pepper to taste
- 2 cloves garlic
- Potatoes 400 gr

Preparation:

To prepare the cream of beans, put the beans to soak in abundant cold water for 12 hours (it would be better if you soaked them the night before leaving them in water overnight). After the soaking time, rinse the beans and drain them. Continuing to make our bean cream, peel and peel the onion and garlic, chop and place them in a pan with melted butter;

add the beans 4, the pinch of cumin and coriander, cover with hot water 6 and let it simmer for about an hour, until the beans have softened, then add salt and pepper.

Take 3/4 of beans, mash them with a fork or blend. Then mix the bean puree with the whole ones; and place the bean cream obtained in 4 individual bowls.

Aside, cook the potatoes in the oven.

Bacon omelet

Ingredients

- 6 eggs
- 150 g of diced bacon
- 100 g of scamorza
- Extra virgin olive oil to taste
- •Salt to taste
- •Pepper as needed

Preparation

Cook the bacon cubes in a non-stick pan with a little extra virgin olive oil for a few minutes, until they are colorful, then transfer them to a plate and set aside temporarily.

In a bowl beat 3 eggs, salt them, pepper them and pour them in the same pan in which you have browned the bacon. Roll the pan slightly to spread the eggs evenly over the entire surface.

Cook the eggs over medium heat for a few minutes and, as soon as they begin to congeal, spread half the bacon and the sliced scarmorza on one half of the omelet, then close it in 2 and continue cooking.

Cook for a few more minutes and, when the omelet is golden on the outside, and the cheese is melted, you can remove it from the pan and keep it aside while you prepare the second.

Serve the omelet hot.

Chicken with parsley and nuts

- chicken
- 1 bunch of parsley
- 2 tbsp walnuts
- 4 tablespoons of olive oil
- 2 cloves of garlic
- 3 tablespoons parmesan or grated pecorino
- Salt and Pepper to Taste.

Put the oil in a saucepan and fry the garlic for two to three minutes. Put the oil aside and let it cool. Finely chop the parsley, washed and dried, with the walnuts and garlic used to flavor the oil. When they are well minced, add the cold oil a little at a time. It must be a compound similar to the Genoese pesto. Add the chicken breast and cook. Serve hot.

Conclusions

According to nutritionists Aidan Goggins and Glen Matten, who have developed the Sirtfood Diet, the consumption of certain foods would activate sirtuins, a group of genes that stimulate the metabolism, burn fat and promote rapid weight loss.

According to the studies developed by the two doctors, these genes stimulate the metabolism, cause fat burning and promote a fairly rapid weight loss. In addition, sirtuins are able to repair cells and improve general health by transforming from slimming instruments to elixirs of longevity.

The genes of thinness, responsible for the repair and rejuvenation of cells, accelerate their activity by drawing on fat reserves and increasing resistance to diseases. The same goal can be achieved without going hungry or by eating Sirt foods. In short, fasting is of little use because the body does not receive the necessary need for nutrients and therefore triggers a series of changes on normal growth processes to survive.

The Sirtfood Diet is based on the inclusion and not on the exclusion of food, which allows you to lose more than 3 kilos in a week without undoable sacrifices. And if some of these are not so well known, most of them are known foods used in traditional cooking.

Obviously, this diet is not a magic potion, but it tries to convey how new studies help us plan a food model capable of making us lose weight by suffering less and aging in a healthy way.

The Sirtfood Diet consists of two phases. Phase 1 guarantees the loss of 3.5 kilos in 7 days and is the one that produces the greatest results. During the first three days, you can eat a maximum of 1000 daily calories divided between three green juices and a solid meal, all based on Sirt foods. From the fourth to the seventh day, the calories will become fifteen hundred. Two green juices and two solid Sirt meals are included daily.

Phase 2 is the maintenance phase and lasts 14 days. During this period, the primary objective will be to consolidate weight loss; however, it will be possible to continue losing weight by continuing to eat plenty of Sirt foods.

Aidan Goggins and Glen Matten ensure that the lost kilograms will not come back to haunt you. In addition, the diet can be followed as needed, when you want to eliminate a few extra kg or centimeters, but not for an extended period. Practicing a little physical activity will certainly do well both during the first and second phases, as with any other diet.

However, before starting a new diet to lose weight, our advice is to have a specialist follow you because psychophysical well-being also passes through a correct and tailor-made diet.

Criticisms

Is the Sirtfood Diet effective? The problem is that there is not much evidence to support it.

In the book "Sirt, the lean gene-diet," the results of a pilot study conducted by the authors and involving 39 participants from their fitness center are presented. However, the results of this study do not appear to have been published elsewhere.

For a week, the participants followed the diet and exercised daily physical activity. At the end of the week, participants lost an average of 3.2

kg and maintained or even gained muscle mass. However, it appears that the method has not been tested and documented in the long term.

Limiting the calorie intake to 1,000 calories, physical training, and the almost total elimination of carbohydrates, followed in the first phase of the Sirtfood Diet, will usually lead to weight loss. Be that as it may, this type of rapid weight loss is neither authentic nor sustainable, and this study did not follow participants after the first week to see if they had gained weight afterward.

In addition, with the Sirtfood Diet, aimed at activating the "weight loss genes", foods that activate the metabolism are assumed, while pretending to be sated, thus creating a sort of deception for the body. This diet is likely to help you lose a few kilograms in the beginning, but you should be very careful not to gain weight once again after the diet is over.

As for disease prevention, three weeks are probably not long enough to have a measurable long-term impact. On the other hand, adding Sirt foods to your usual long-term diet can be a good idea. In this case, however, it is not recommended to follow the diet for long-term periods, but instead to follow the Sirtfood Diet and continue with a personalized one, rich in Sirt foods.